In Honor of

Gary "Papa Bear" Ewing

8/17/1953-2/1/2024

Daddy-dillo is a talented and creative armadillo. He likes to use jokes to make the other animals laugh and comes up with fun ideas that all of the animals love. He knows just how to help others shine their brightest!

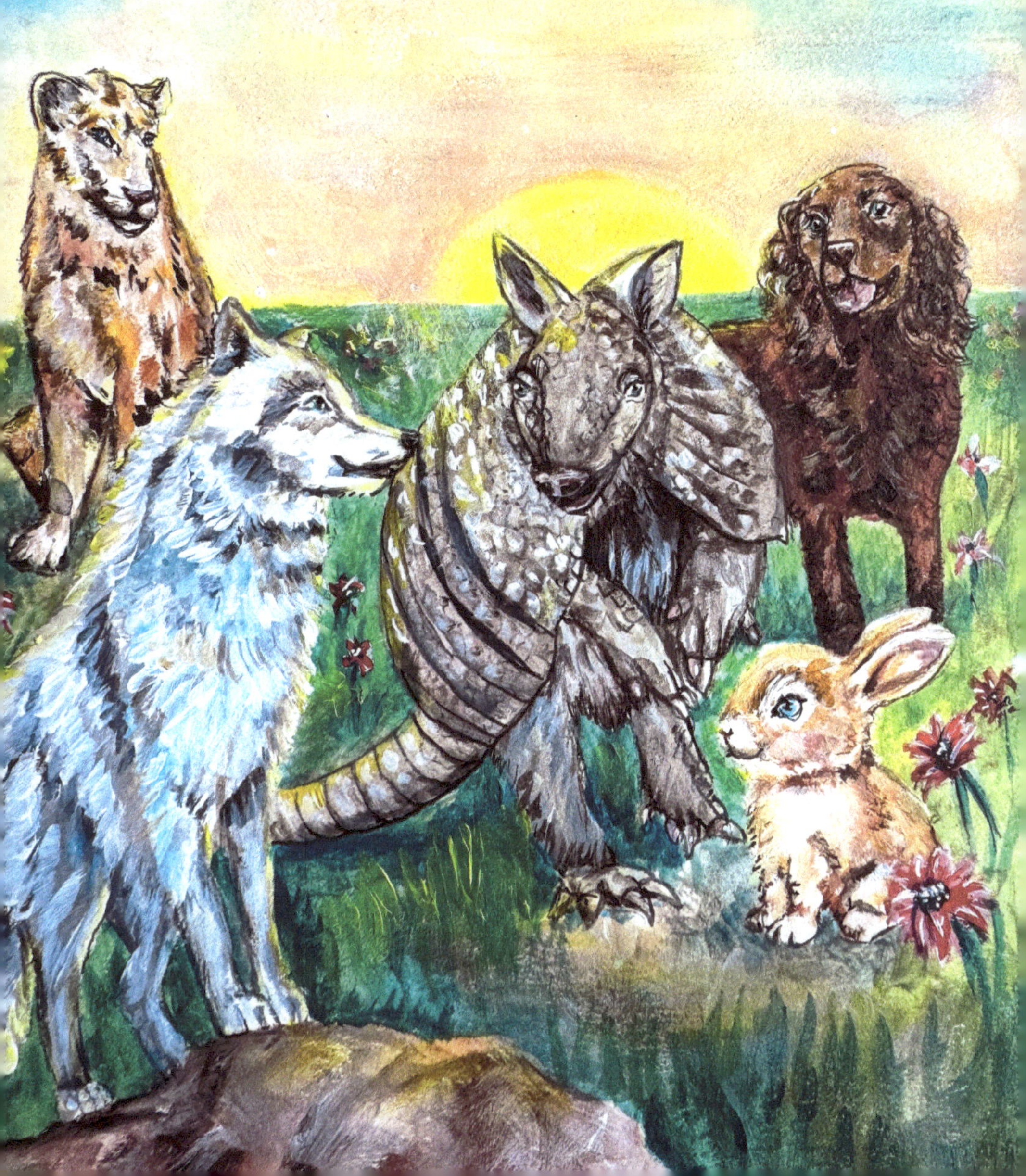

But sometimes Daddy-dillo's brain feels Mixed Up and doesn't work the way he wants it to. Sometimes he doesn't feel happy, even when fun things are happening. Other times he can't feel calm, even when he's not sure what he's worried about. Sometimes Daddy-dillo's brain gets so Mixed Up he can feel down for months and even though the other animals try to help him, he might think he needs to be alone.

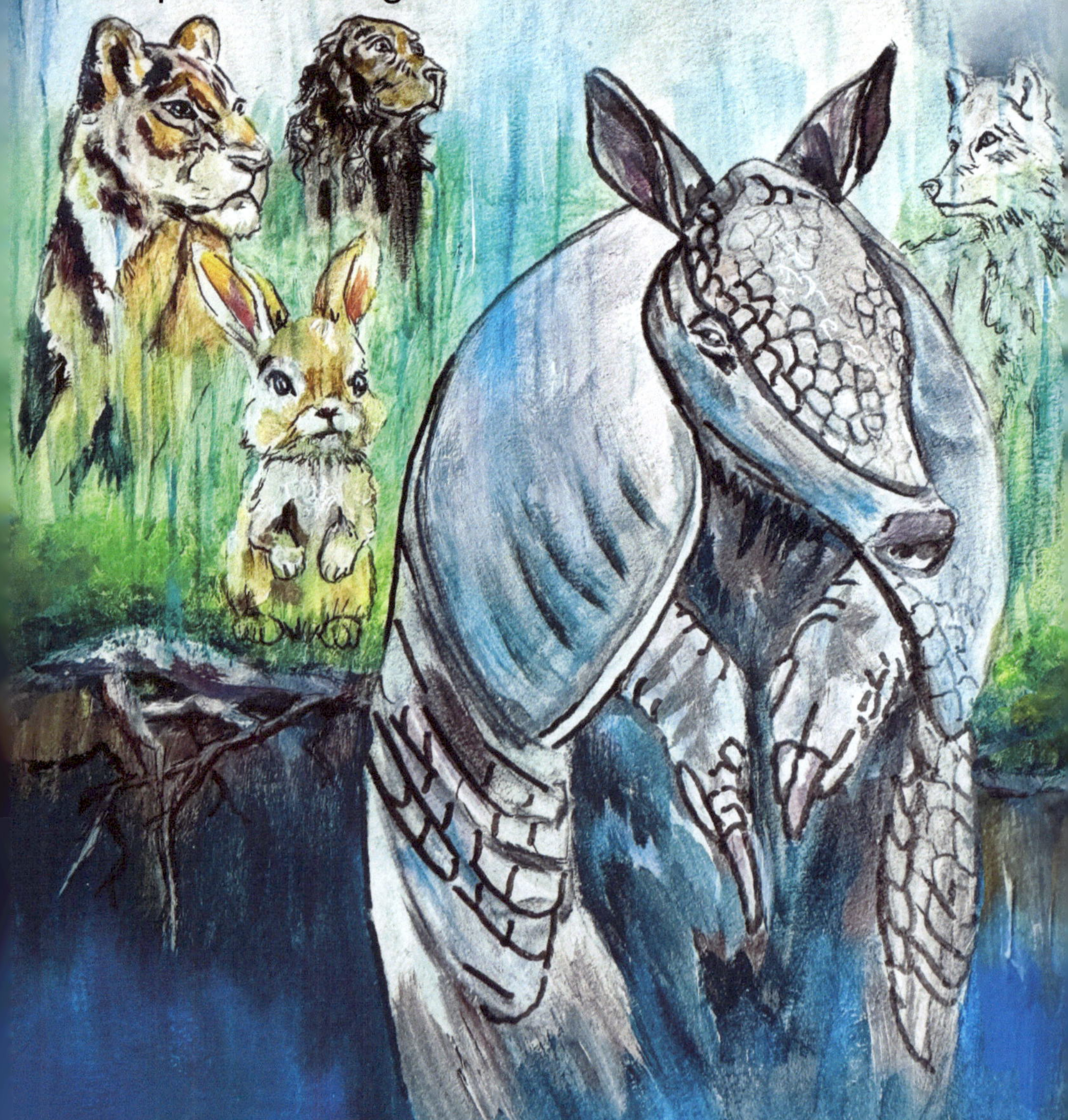

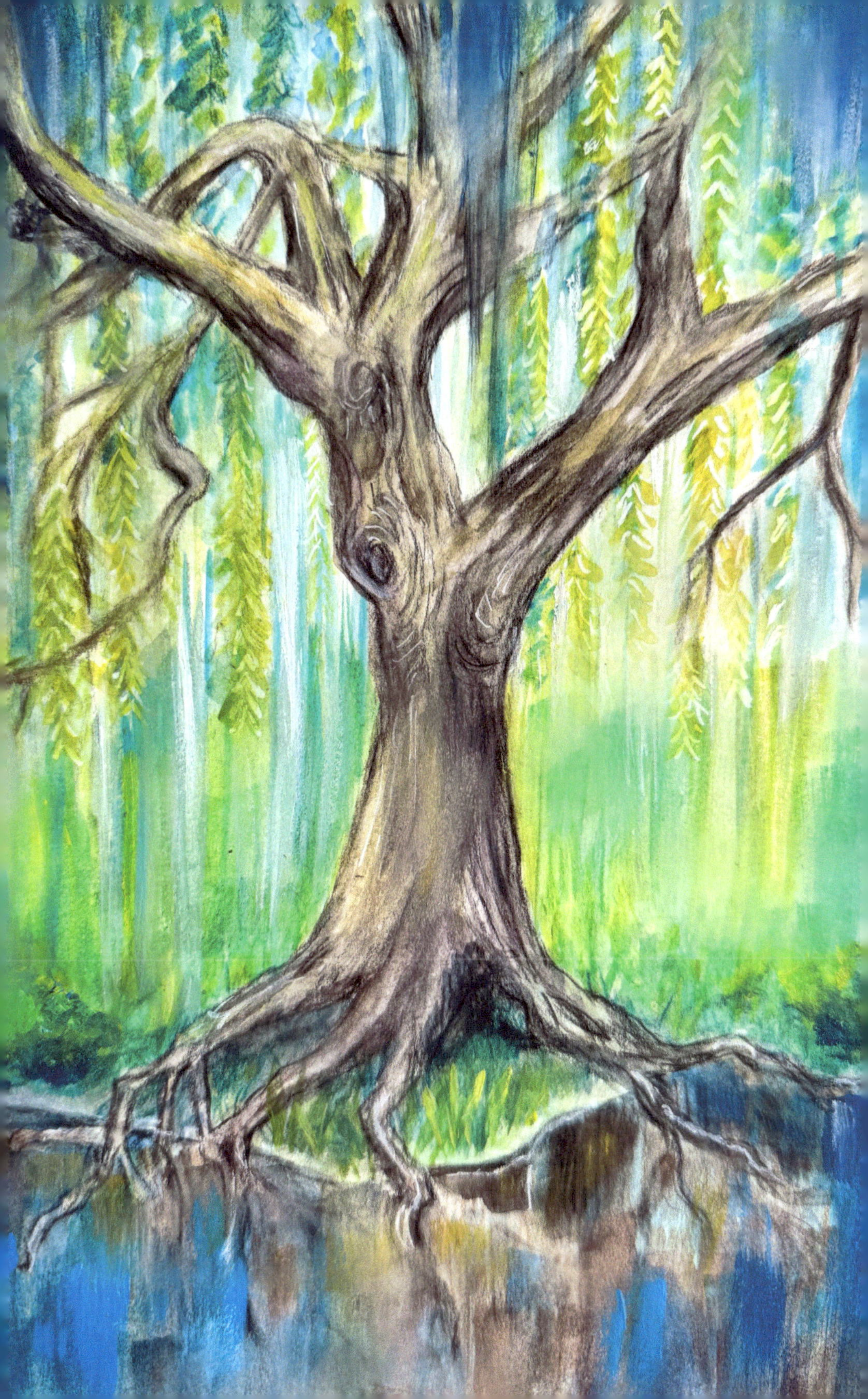

"Maybe if I buy all of the things I want, I will feel better," says Daddy-dillo and he buys lots of new, fun things.

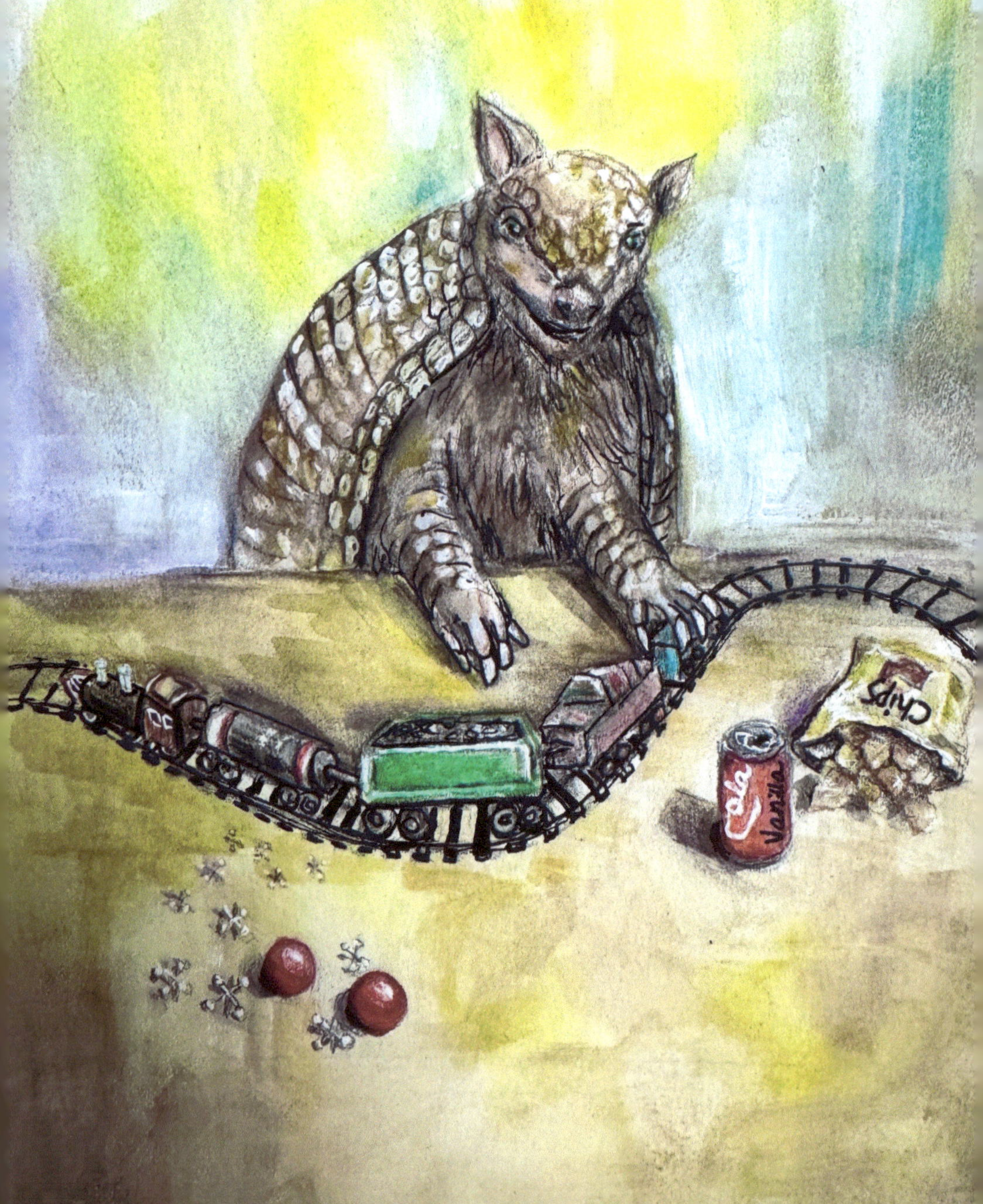

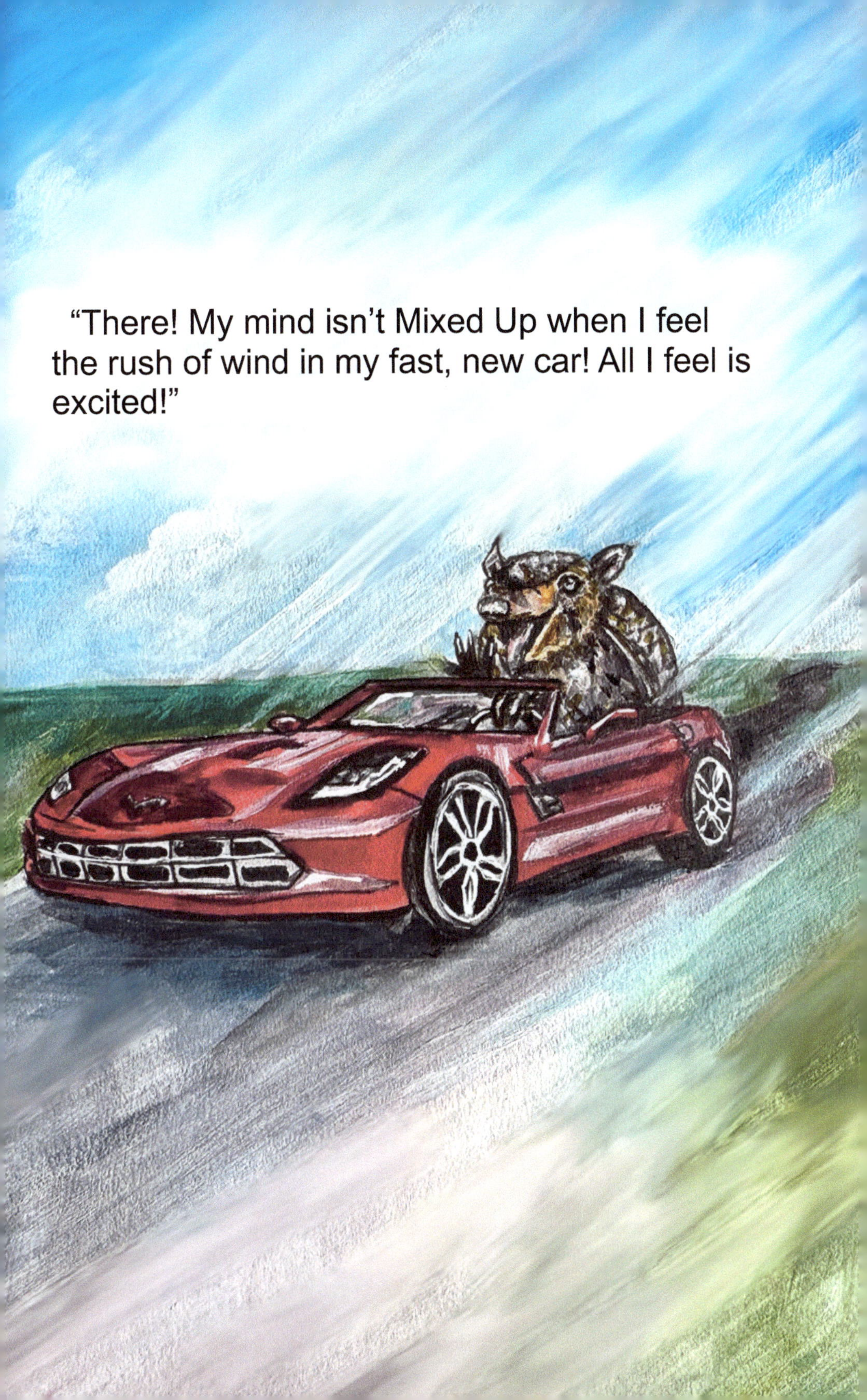

"There! My mind isn't Mixed Up when I feel the rush of wind in my fast, new car! All I feel is excited!"

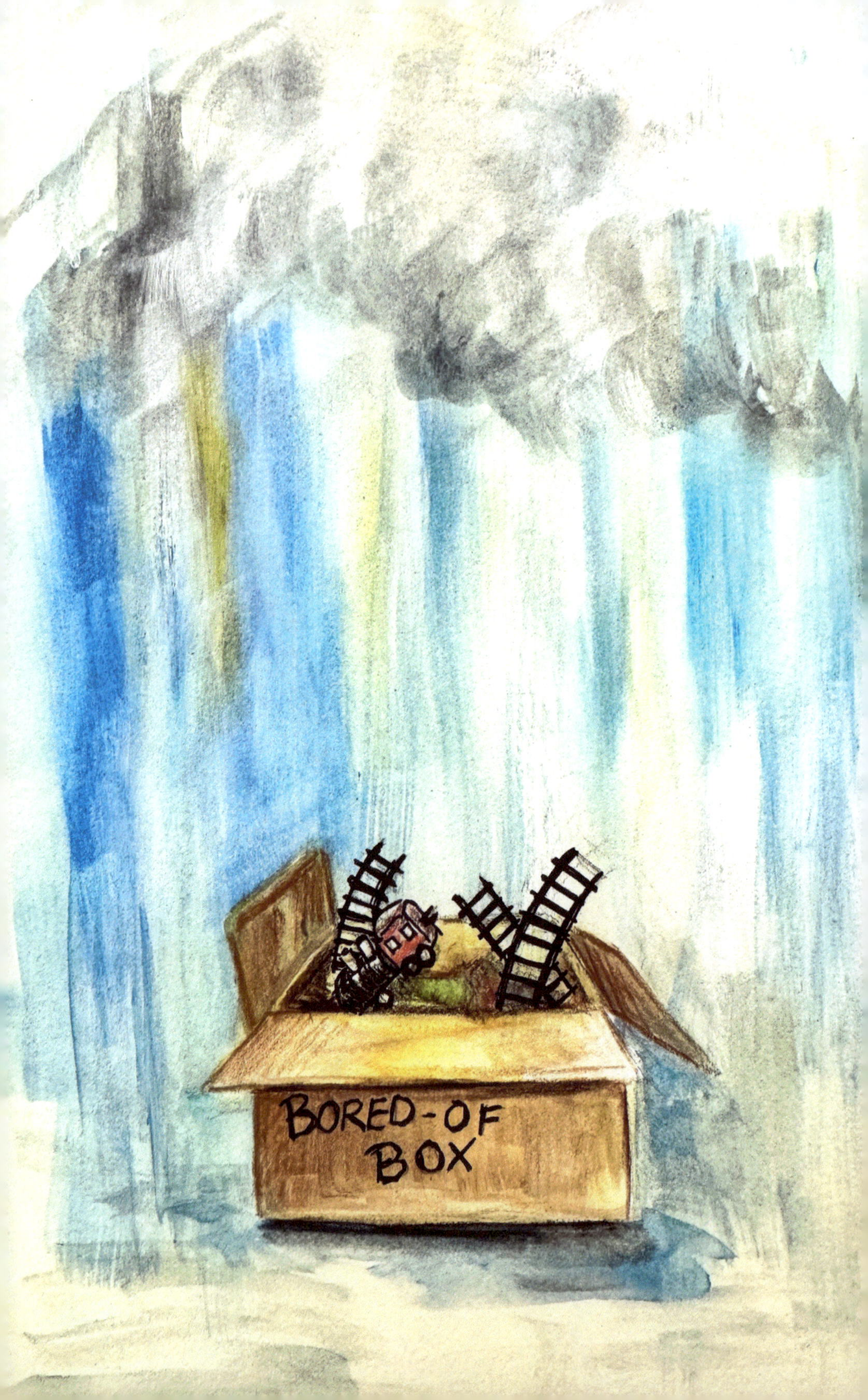
BORED-OF
BOX

But new fancy things only stay fun for a short while. "I got the things I wanted, so why doesn't it feel good enough? My mind still feels Mixed Up."

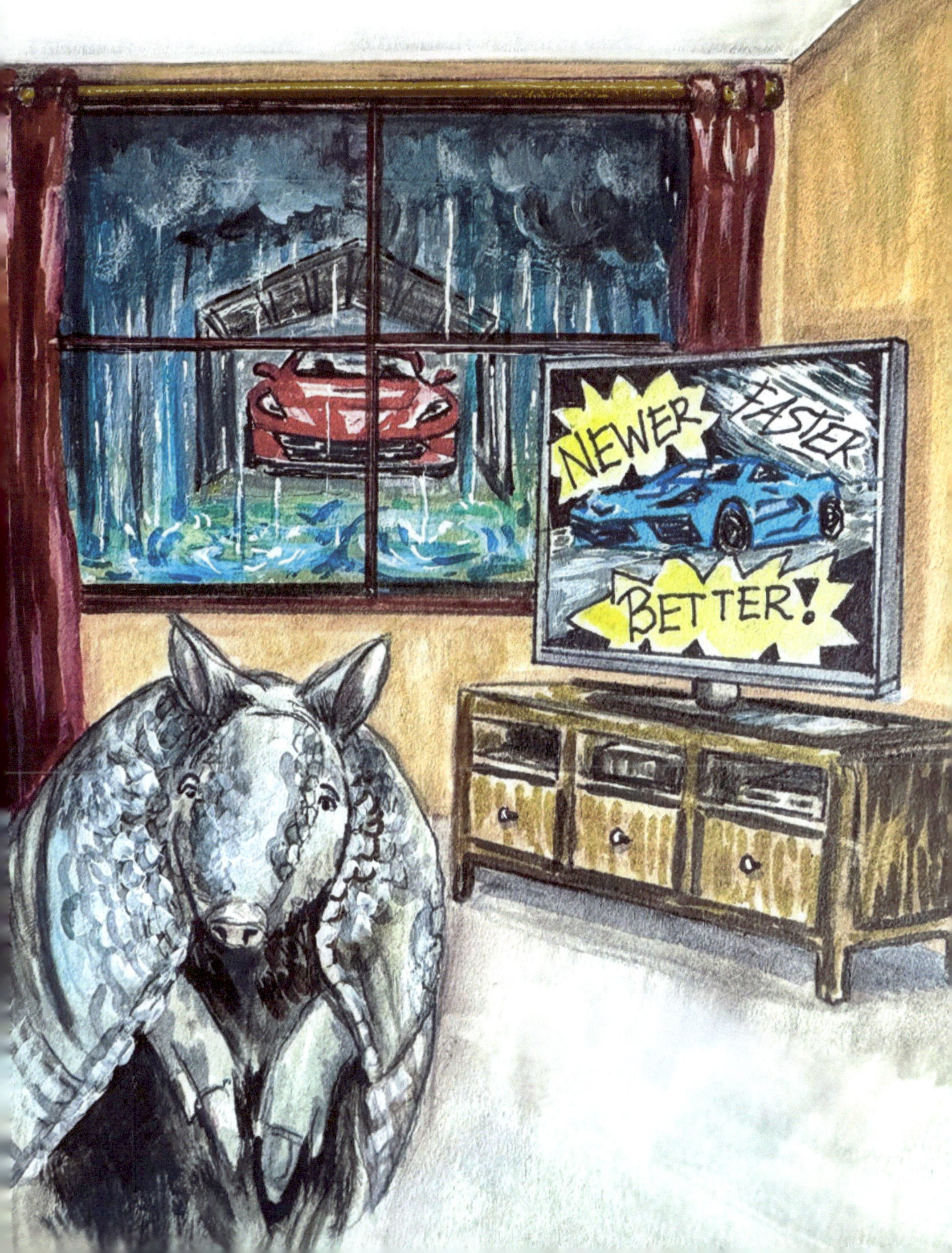

Kate Spaniel tries to help Daddy-dillo in the best way she knows. "Let me plan your day with things that will make you feel better. I'll set times for you to have fun, exercise, eat healthy foods, and relax." It sounds good, but Daddy-dillo's mind gets Mixed Up and tells him, "All that is too hard. Do what you want, when you want and that will be easier!"

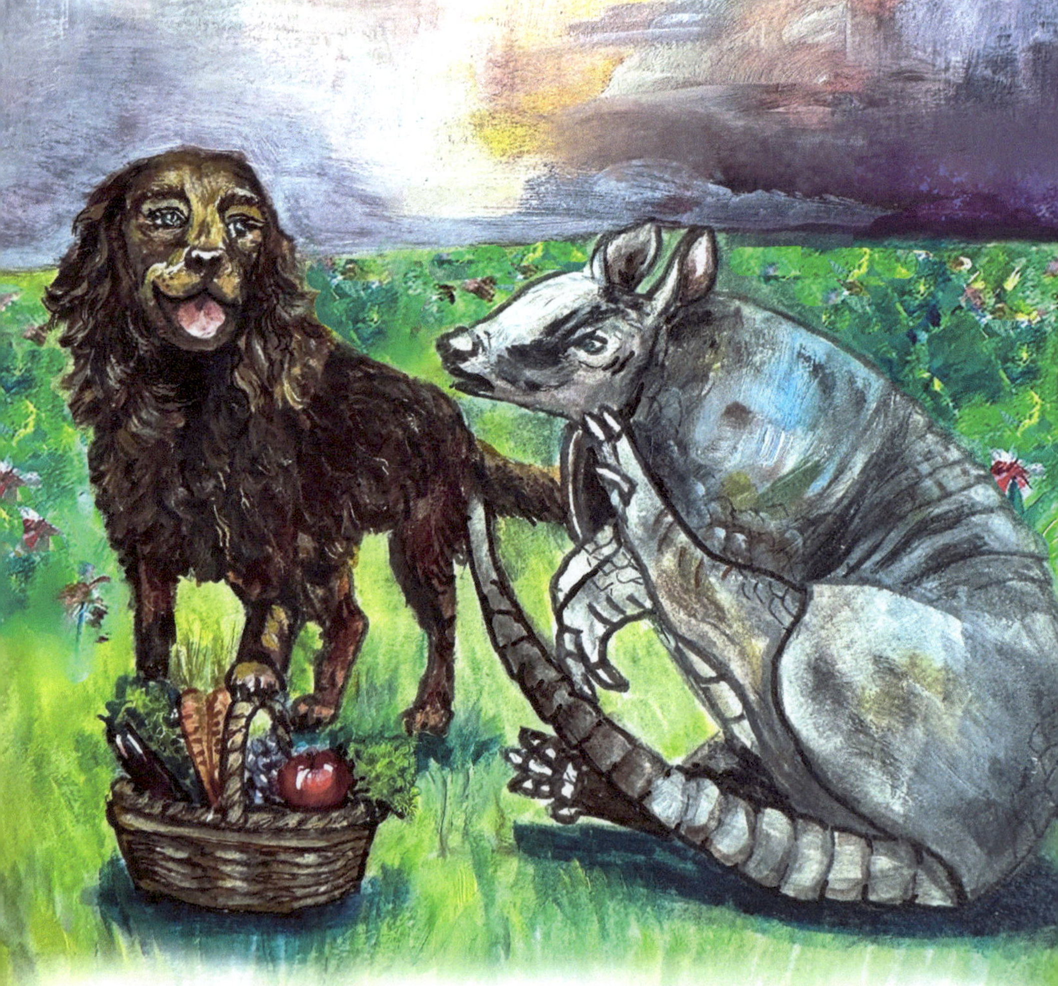

"I'm not capable of changing my habits," Daddy-dillo argues, and soon his body starts to feel sick.

Kate Spaniel feels frustrated as she leaves. Then Mother Earth speaks to her from the sky, "Kate Spaniel, you can't change others or make them do more than they are able…

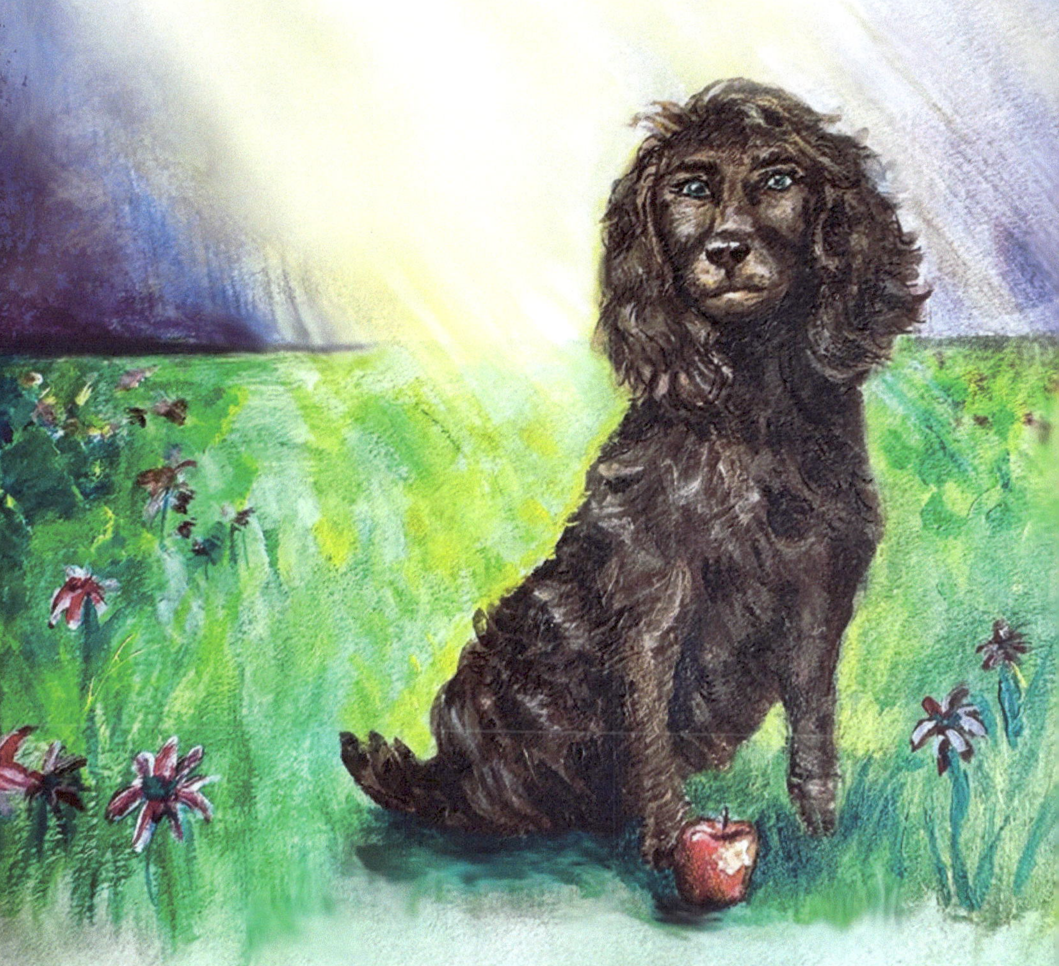

Keep your healthy habits with pride as you see how helpful they are. You have not failed if you can not fix or control what is in someone else's mind."

Some days, Daddy-dillo wants to sleep for the entire day and miss out on all of the activities the other animals are doing. "I can cheer you up," says Baby Bunny, "I will tell you kind words and funny stories if you just pay attention to me!"

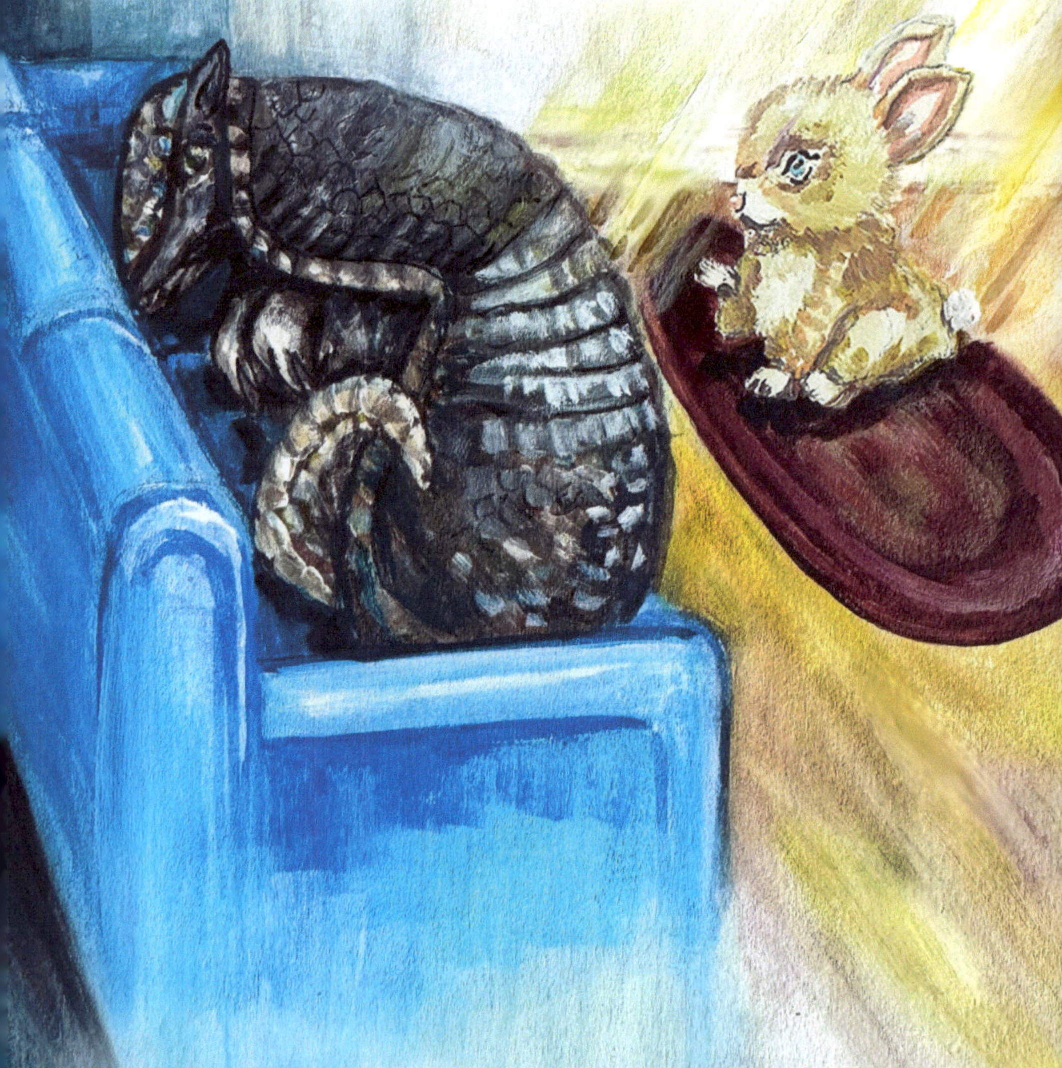

Daddy-dillo's heart smiles and wants to believe Baby Bunny, but listening to his Mixed Up mind has worn him out. "Some other time," Daddy-dillo says, and rolls back over to sleep.

Mother Earth speaks to Baby Bunny, "He heard you, but sometimes when a mind feels Mixed Up, it might not be ready to be cheered up. You are still lovable and worthy of being listened to. Never lose your kind smile."

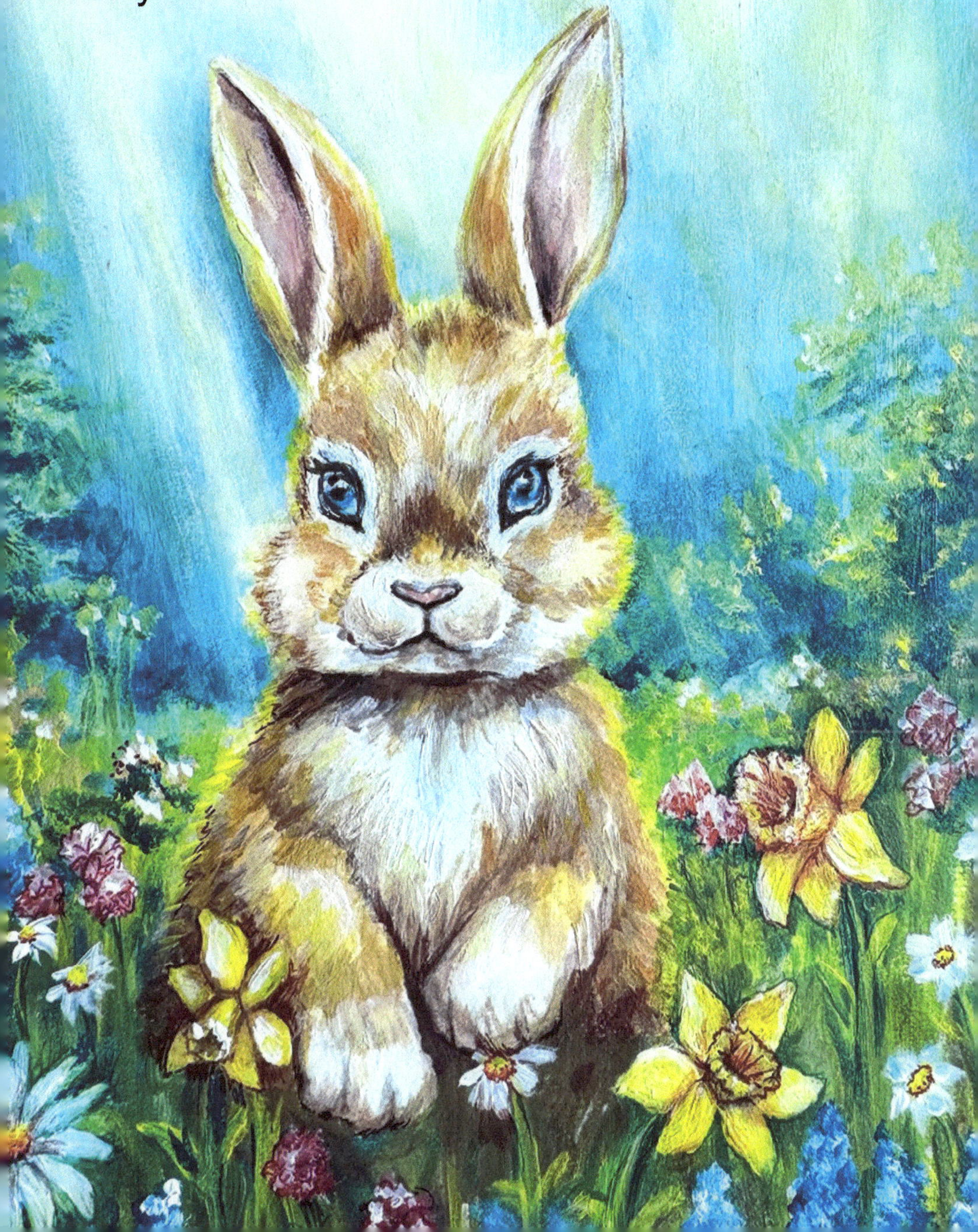

Daddy-dillo's mind begins to feel so Mixed Up he stops trying. He stops taking care of the things he owns and his body gets sicker. Brother Wolf comes to help around the house and speaks encouraging words to him, but pride and shame keep him from praising Brother Wolf's help.

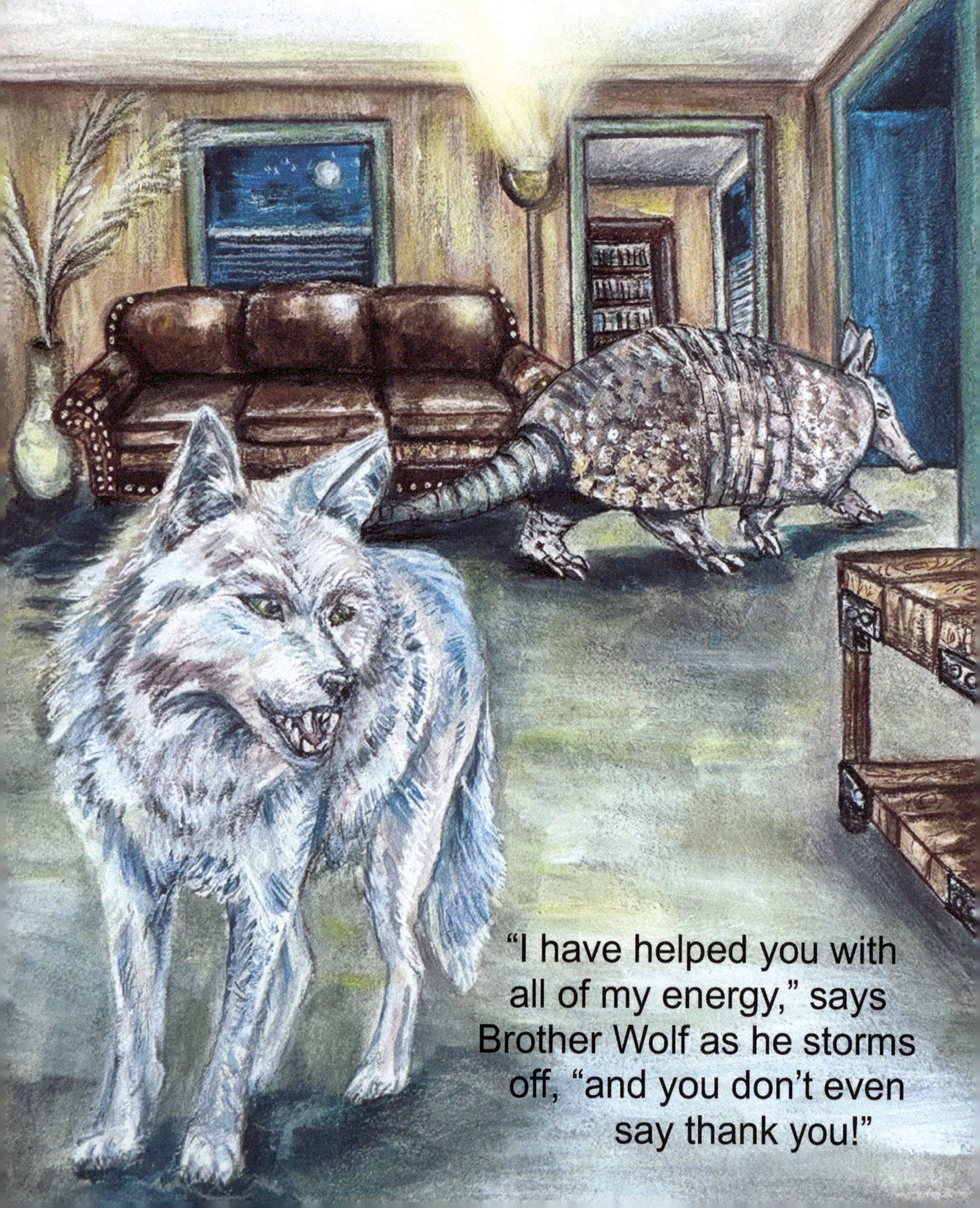

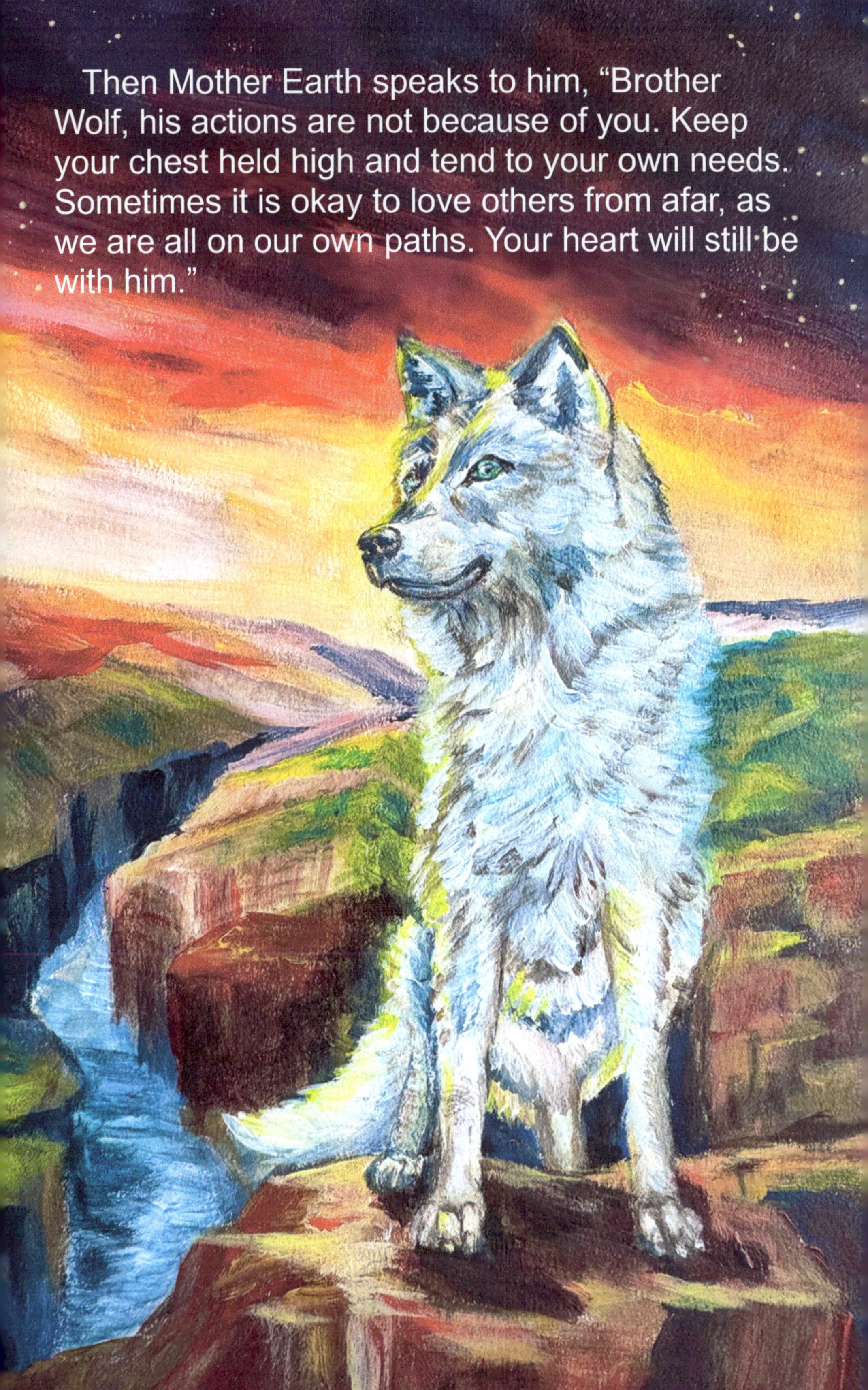

Then Mother Earth speaks to him, "Brother Wolf, his actions are not because of you. Keep your chest held high and tend to your own needs. Sometimes it is okay to love others from afar, as we are all on our own paths. Your heart will still be with him."

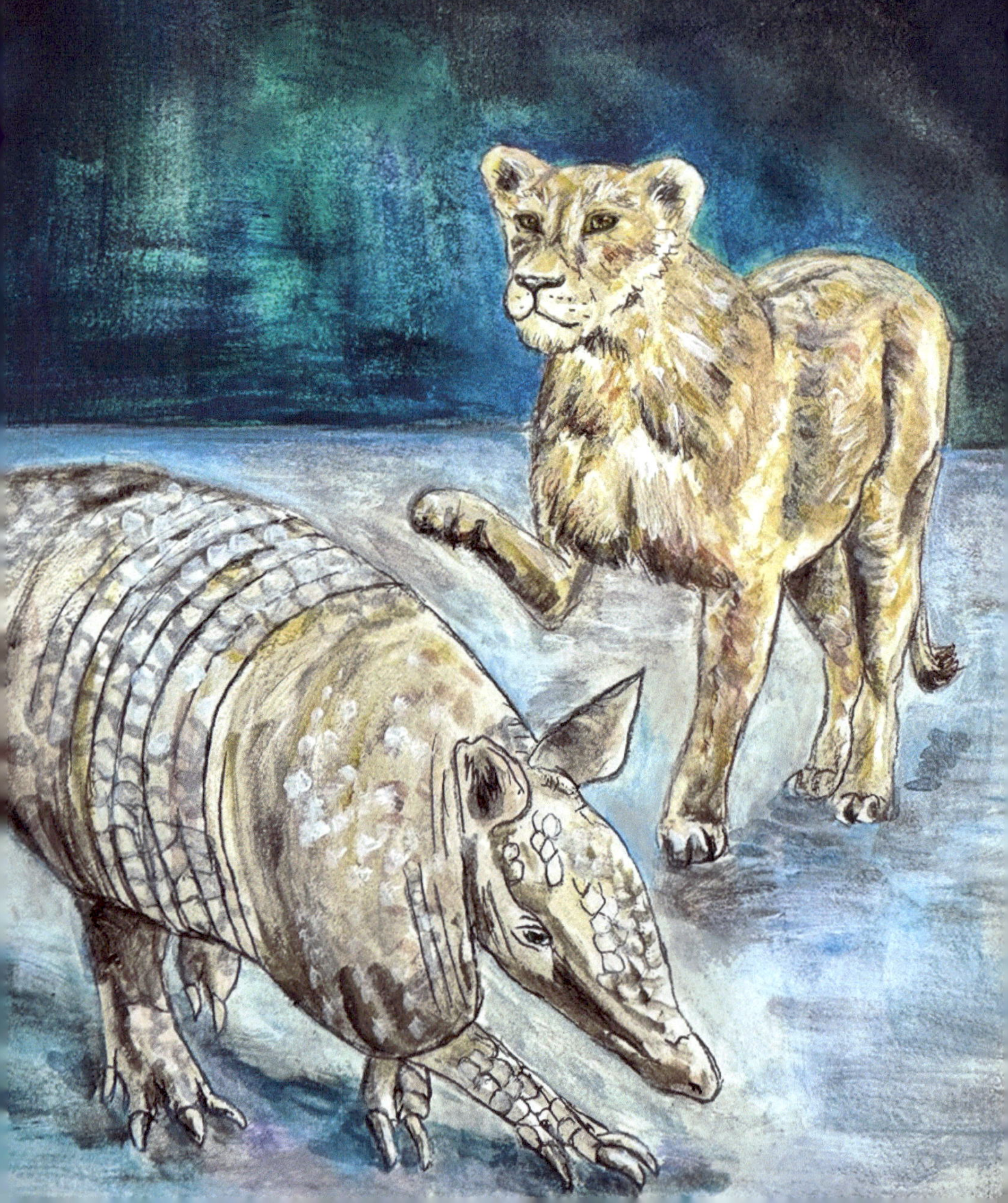

"I've pushed away those who love me," Daddy-dillo says sadly to his friend, Lionness. She tells him, "*Who you are* is not your Mixed Up mind. It's never too late to learn how to manage it. You should talk to a counselor regularly and a doctor may have you take medicine."

Daddy-dillo agrees and a doctor has him try
a blue medicine, but it makes him very sleepy.

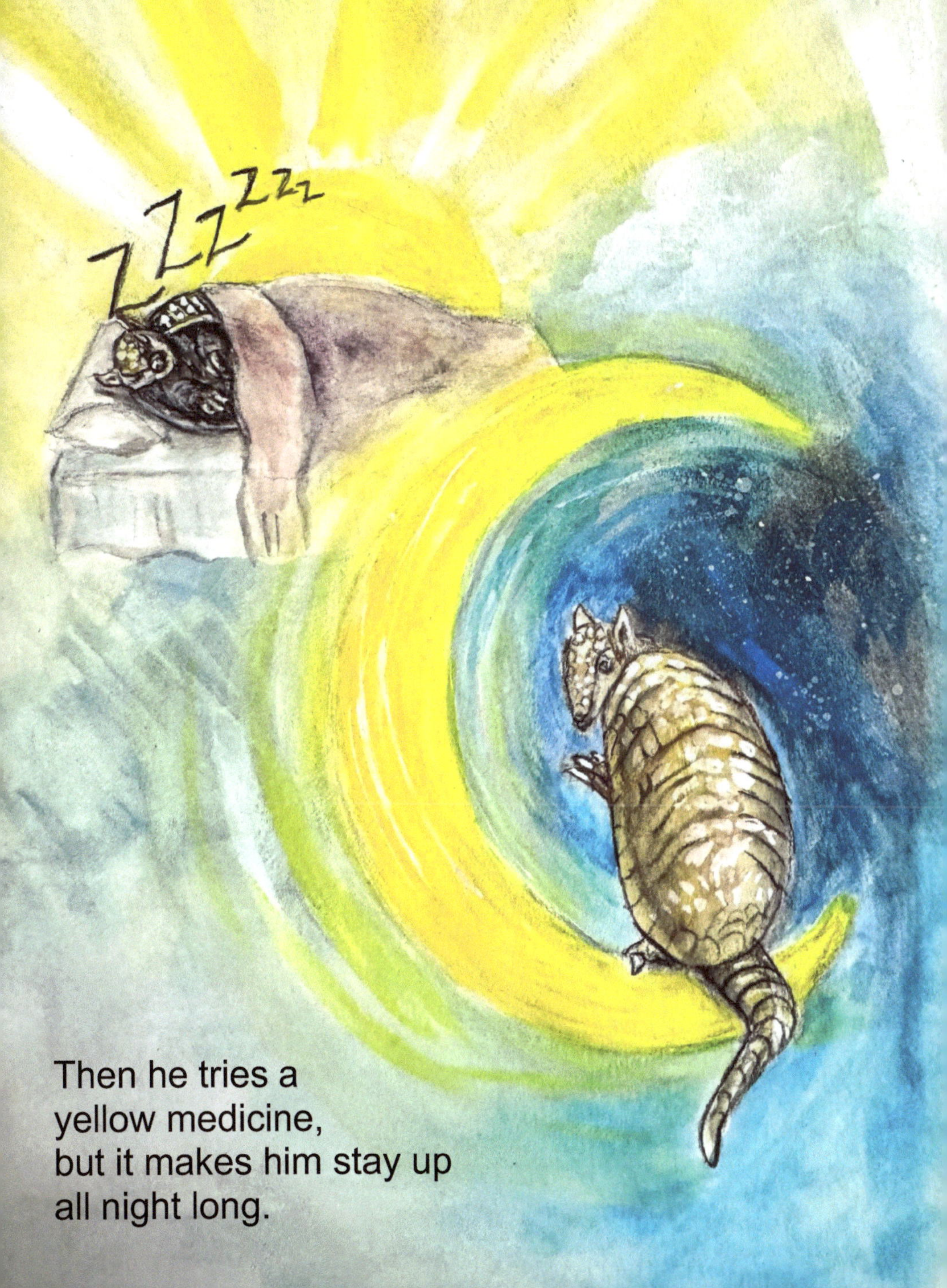

Then he tries a
yellow medicine,
but it makes him stay up
all night long.

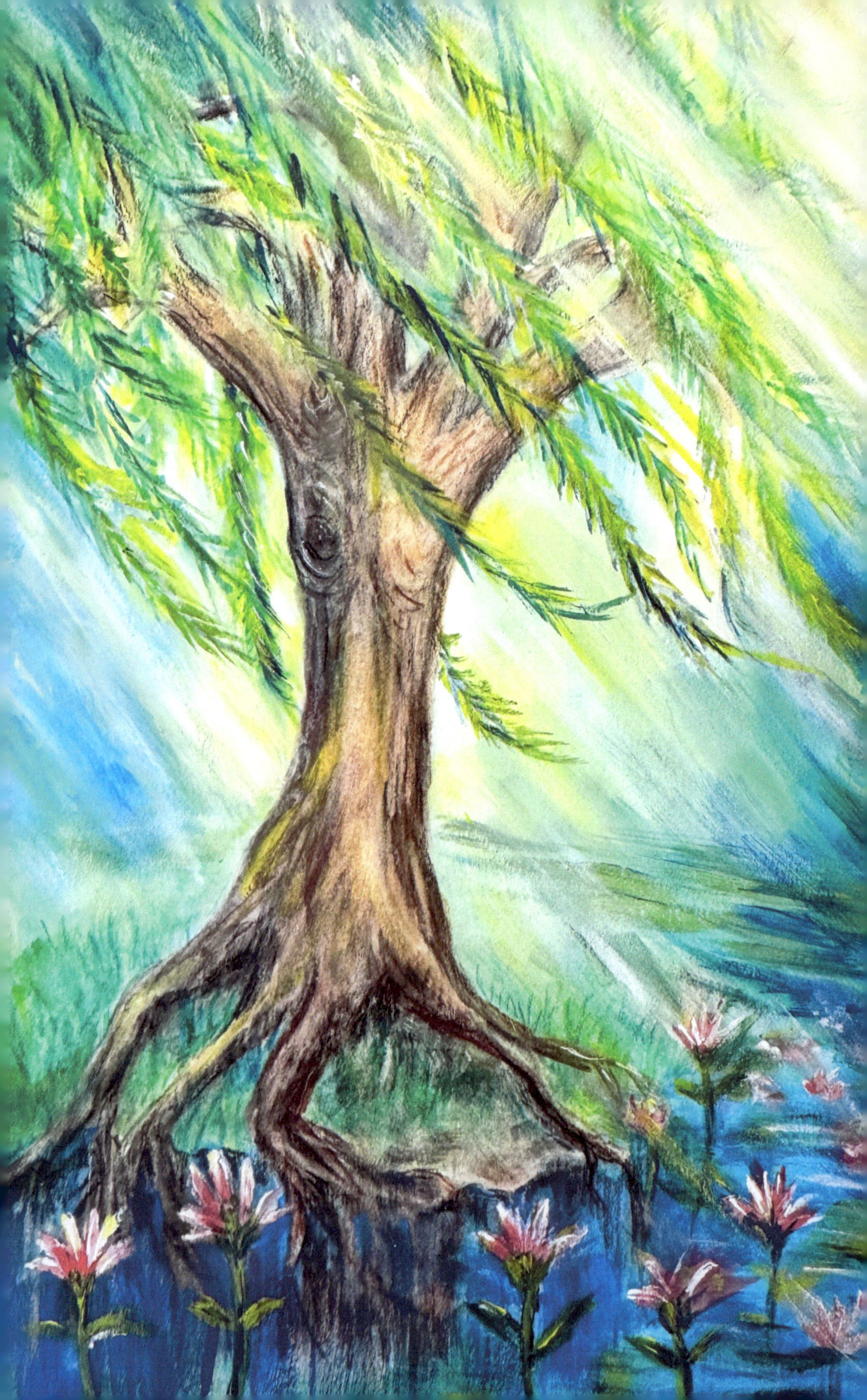

Then he tries a white medicine, and it seems to help him control his Mixed Up mind! His brain still feels Mixed Up sometimes, but he shares his thoughts with a counselor and learns he doesn't have to believe everything the Mixed Up thoughts say. Daddy-dillo practices being kind to himself, "If I can help others shine so brightly, why can't I make myself shine too?"

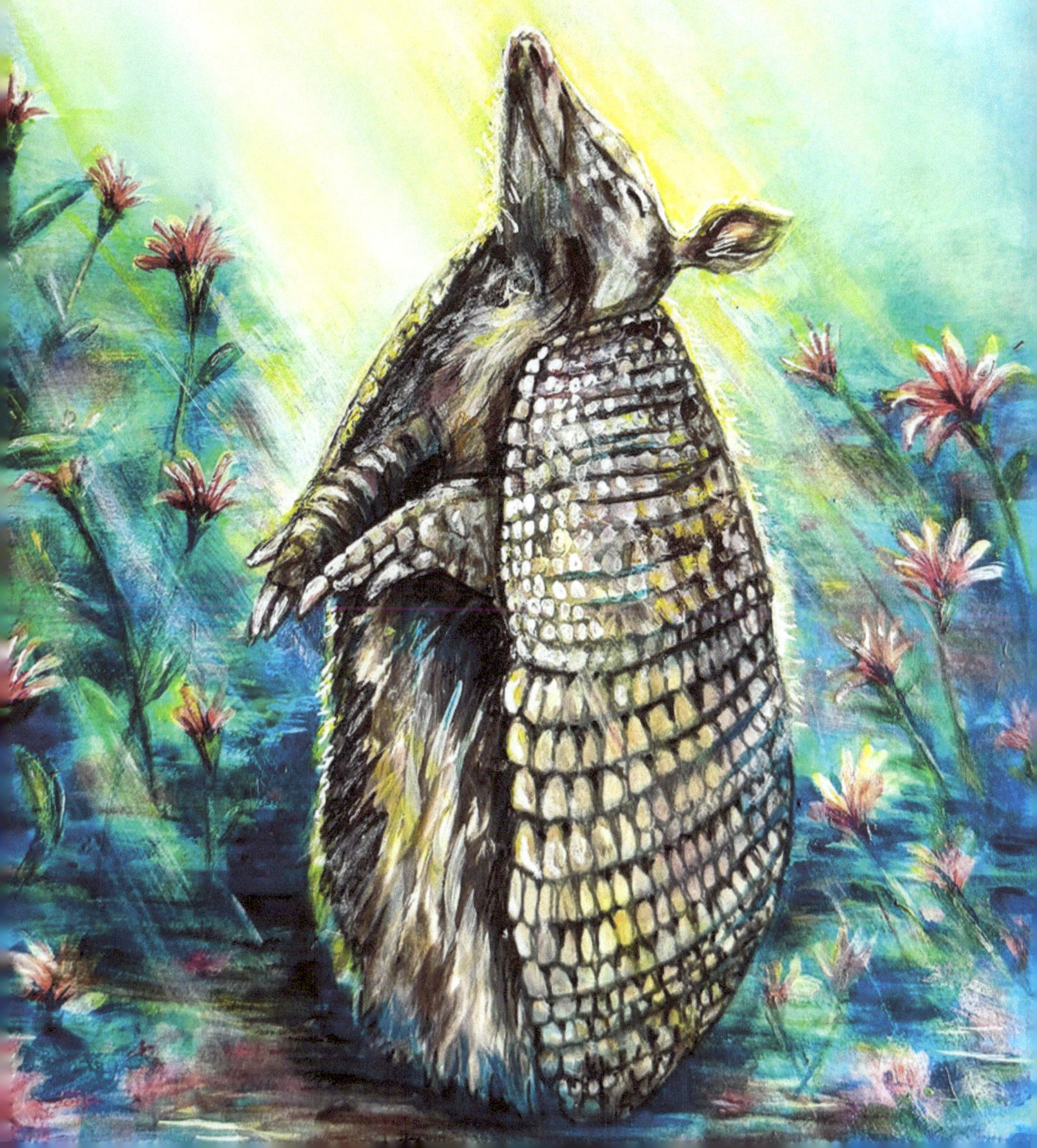

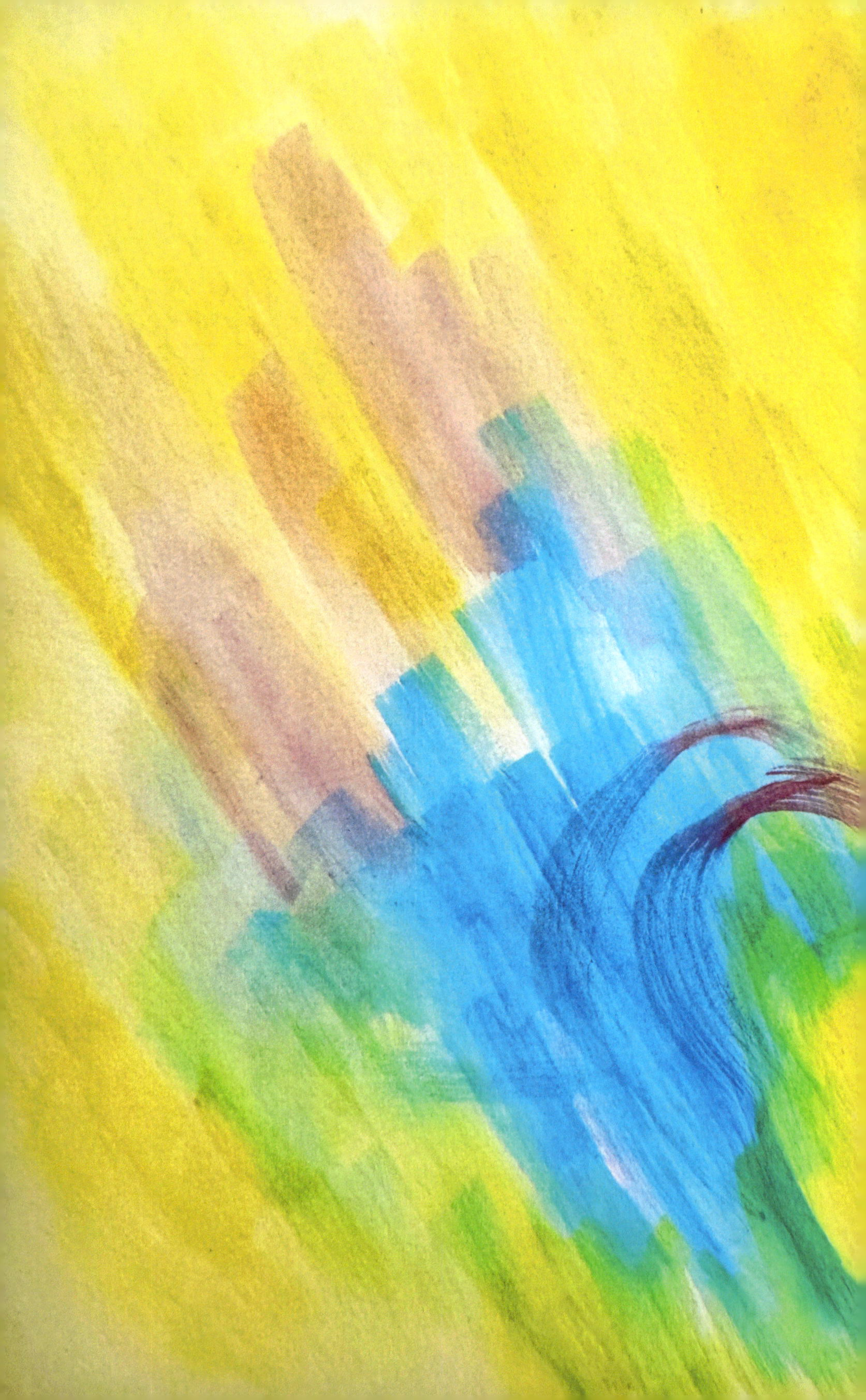

Daddy-dillo never wanted to push away those he loved or make them feel rejected. He tells the other animals, "My Mixed Up mind has nothing to do with any of you, your worth, or how much I love you- for the love I have for you all is deep and true. Please don't let my actions make you feel any less about yourselves. Let's enjoy this moment while my mind isn't so Mixed Up."

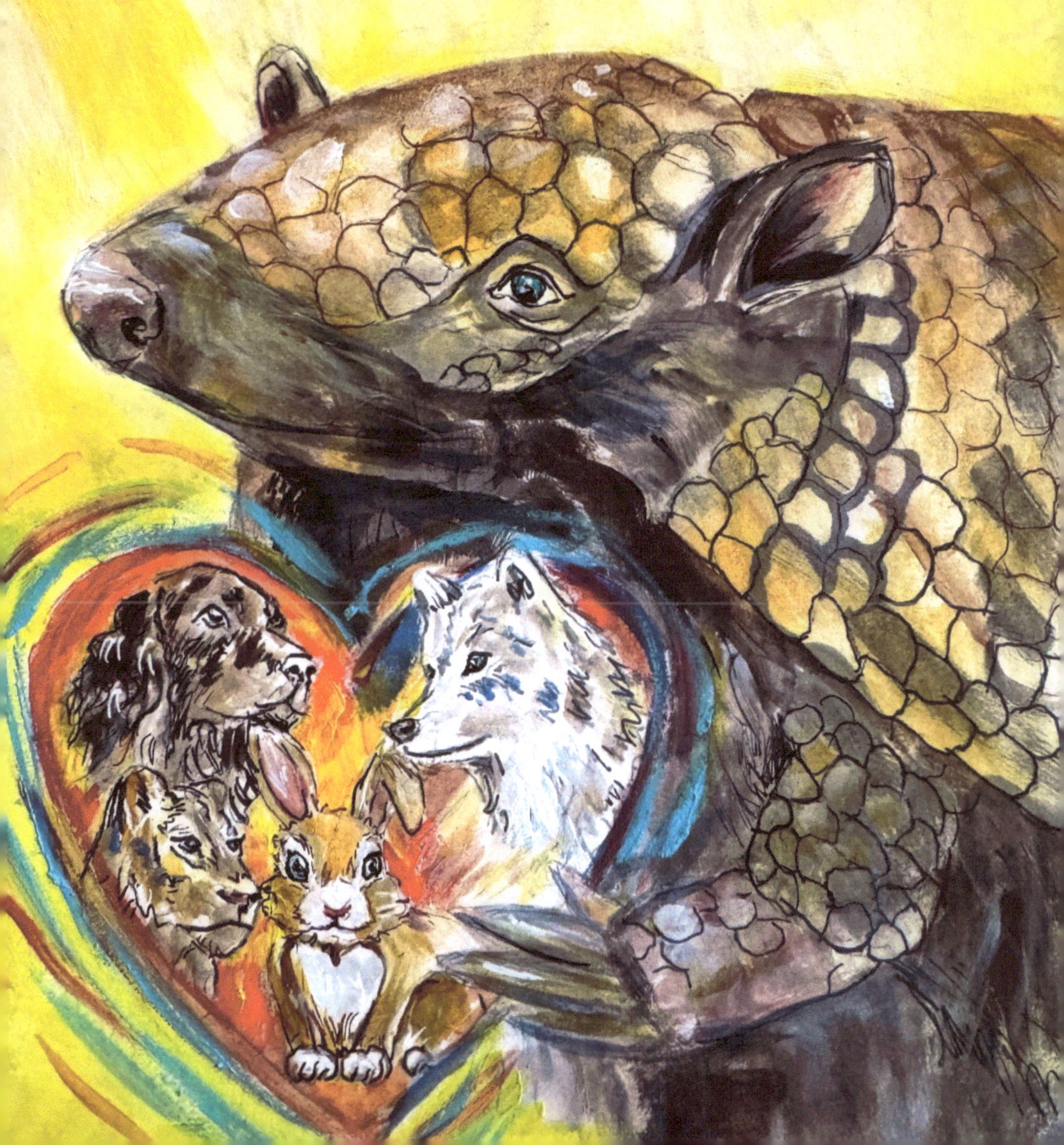

Dear Reader,

Having a loved one with mental illness, like Daddy-dillo, can be challenging and confusing, but it is nothing to be ashamed of as it is very common. While there are many different types of mental illnesses, Daddy-dillo simply calls his mind "Mixed Up" whenever he feels like his thoughts don't match up with how he thinks they should. Like many parents with mental illness, Daddy-dillo is loving and has many wonderful qualities, but inside his mind, he deals with feeling sad, alone, or sometimes anxious for long periods of time. This can make it hard to think clearly, accept help from others, or stick to healthy habits.

Remember to take care of yourself first, ask another adult, teacher, or counselor for help when needed, and understand that you are not alone. Sometimes a parent may not be able to manage his/her mental illness and it is important to know that it has nothing to do with you- it's not your fault or your responsibility to fix someone else. There is hope, though, as millions of people around the world successfully manage their mental health every day.

Best wishes,

Brittany, the Baby Bunny

www.ingramcontent.com/pod-product-compliance
Lightning Source LLC
Chambersburg PA
CBHW041805260726
48664CB00034B/428